First Steps in
Vesico-Vaginal Fistula
Repair

To Dr Catherine Hamlin and the staff of the Addis Ababa Fistula Hospital – especially to Mamitu Gashe, the patient turned surgeon

First Steps in Vesico-Vaginal Fistula Repair

Brian Hancock MD FRCS
Honorary Consultant Surgeon
University Hospital of South Manchester, Manchester, UK

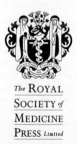

The ROYAL
SOCIETY *of*
MEDICINE
PRESS *Limited*

© 2005 Royal Society of Medicine Press Ltd

Published by the Royal Society of Medicine Press Ltd
1 Wimpole Street, London W1G 0AE, UK
Tel: +44 (0)20 7290 2921
Fax: +44 (0)20 7290 2929
Email: publishing@rsm.ac.uk
Website: www.rsmpress.co.uk

British Library Cataloguing in Publication Data
A catalogue record for this book is available from the British Library

ISBN 1-85315-611-6

This publication is supported by educational grants from the Hamlin Churchill Childbirth Injuries Fund (UK charity no 237741; www.charitynet.org/~HCCIF) and the Uganda Childbirth Injuries Fund (UK charity no 10991354).

Distribution in Europe and Rest of World:

Marston Book Services Ltd
PO Box 269
Abingdon
Oxon OX14 4YN, UK
Tel: +44 (0)1235 465500
Fax: +44 (0)1235 465555
Email: direct.order@marston.co.uk

Distribution in the USA and Canada:

Royal Society of Medicine Press Ltd
c/o Jamco Distribution Inc
1401 Lakeway Drive
Lewisville, TX 75057, USA
Tel: +1 800 538 1287
Fax: +1 972 353 1303
Email: jamco@majors.com

Distribution in Australia and New Zealand:

Elsevier Australia
30-52 Smidmore Street
Marrikville NSW 2204, Australia
Tel: +61 2 9517 8999
Fax: +61 2 9517 2249
Email: service@elsevier.com.au

Typeset by Phoenix Photosetting, Chatham, Kent
Printed in the Netherlands by Alfabase, Alphen aan den Rijn

CONTENTS

Foreword   *vi*
Preface   *vii*

1   Introduction   1

2   Understanding the cause and nature of vesico-vaginal fistulae   3

3   Conservative management of early cases   8

4   Selection of cases for the beginner   10

5   Diagnosis   14

6   Preoperative preparation   19

7   In theatre   21

8   A simple fistula repair, step by step   25

9   Problems and difficulties   31

10 Taking it further   33

11 Repair of anal sphincter injuries   44

12 Postoperative care of the fistula patient   46

13 Comparison of two approaches to fistula repair   55

    Appendix: Books, articles and videos   56
    Acknowledgements   58
    Index   61

FOREWORD

Maternal health is one of the few parameters in international public health that has not changed in recent times. In spite of programmes such as the Safe Motherhood Initiative, little impact has been made on maternal and reproductive health in the developing world.

Improving maternal health is the fifth Millennium Development Goal proposed by the United Nations, to be achieved by 2015. This includes a reduction in maternal mortality by three-quarters relative to 1990. There is still a long way to travel before the goal is reached.

Brian Hancock's book on the management of simple obstetric fistulae is therefore particularly welcome at this time. Even if we cannot improve maternal mortality straight away, one thing that can be done immediately is to repair the damage resulting from obstructed labour. In the past, in spite of the pioneering work of James Marion Sims in Alabama in the 19th century, women who developed a fistula were left to suffer in silence, often isolated and ostracized by family and society. From the middle of the 20th century, thanks to Reg and Catherine Hamlin in Addis Ababa, the problem has become increasingly recognized and treated successfully.

However, fistula surgery is still considered a specialist domain, and there are still far too few specialist centres to cope with the demand. In addition, the problem is largely one that occurs in rural areas as a result of inappropriate management of labour without access to medical care. Patients who develop a fistula can often ill afford either the cost of travel to a specialist centre, or the charges for accommodation and surgery.

This book shows that with appropriate selection, many fistulae can be cured locally, without sophisticated equipment or specialist surgeons. More difficult cases should be referred on, but if the recommendations made here are followed, many women will have their lives improved dramatically without needing to travel to a specialist centre.

Brian Hancock has taught and encouraged many surgeons and gynaecologists to become interested in fistula work. He is known from Ethiopia to Sierra Leone, and has set up a centre to treat injuries from childbirth in Uganda. Since an obstetric fistula is almost unheard of in developed countries, doctors in Europe and America may be unfamiliar with the different appearances and techniques of repair. This book is therefore equally useful for all doctors, whatever their background, when confronted with an obstetric fistula.

Richard Kerr-Wilson, FRCS(Ed), FRCOG
Consultant Obstetrician and Gynaecologist

PREFACE

This publication has been produced as a supplement to the journal *Tropical Doctor*. As many of this journal's readers are physicians, it is hoped that they will pass this publication on to their surgical colleagues, who might not have realized that fistula surgery is not always as difficult as it is commonly perceived.

Almost every African country and other poor countries have thousands of silent sufferers with vesico-vaginal fistula. Fistula surgery does not belong to any one specialty. Anyone with good surgical skills and knowledge of pelvic anatomy can learn to repair the easier cases.

This publication is particularly directed at the postgraduate obstetric and gynaecology student, because practical aspects of fistula management are often omitted from their training.

It is very difficult to find a place for formal training in fistula surgery, and in practice many well-motivated doctors, in either government or independent hospitals, have taught themselves using the scanty teaching material available. It is hoped that this publication will be the stimulus for more doctors to take up fistula surgery, if only for the simpler cases. Small independent hospitals often provide the ideal setting for the practice of fistula repair.

It is hard to imagine any surgery, when successful, that is more rewarding for the patient and surgeon. To give a young woman a new start in life using basic surgical skills has its own very special rewards.

This publication has been sponsored by the Hamlin Churchill Childbirth Injuries Fund and the Uganda Childbirth Injuries Fund.

BH

1   INTRODUCTION

Nobody knows how many patients with vesico-vaginal fistulae there are who have been forgotten and are without hope. Estimates are up to 2 000 000 in Africa alone. In Ethiopia, it is estimated that there are 9000 new cases a year. Fistula repair has a reputation for being difficult, but 25% are quite easy and could be repaired by any competent surgeon with a little instruction.

The purpose of this publication is to help the beginner to get started by recognizing the easy cases and to show step by step how they should be repaired. Postoperative care is described and shown to be very simple.

A doctor with good basic surgical skills and some initiative could make a tremendous impact by repairing these simpler cases.

A recent survey of fistula repair throughout Uganda revealed that only 270 repairs were carried out in 2002, the vast majority by visiting fistula experts. Why were so few being done by local surgeons? Reasons given were:

- There was a perceived view that fistula surgery is difficult.
- The results were thought to be poor.
- There was no opportunity to learn fistula surgery.
- There was a lack of special instruments and equipment.
- No specialist nursing care was available.

Some fistula operations are very difficult, and even experts cannot cure every case. The most experienced surgeons claim that 95% of fistulae can be closed (but they have to operate on 10% a second or third time to achieve this figure). However, closure of the fistula does not always mean that the patient will be dry. Another 15% or more will have severe stress incontinence because the urethra and bladder have been so badly damaged. A few may improve, but for those who do not, the operation has failed. Secondary operations for stress are possible, but have uncertain results.

A reasonably experienced surgeon who takes on all the cases that he or she sees can at best probably only make 75% of cases really dry. Of course, the surgeon who turns down the difficult cases will have much better results. For the simple cases described in this account, a near 100% success rate should be possible. This explains the paradox that the better one is at repairing fistulae, the worse are the results, because the expert rarely turns anyone away.

The following points are of note:

- No special instruments or equipment are needed to cure the simple cases.
- Postoperative nursing is important but is not complicated.

I know of no other condition where such a variety exists from the simplest case, which can be completed in half an hour, to the most difficult, which will defeat the most experienced surgeon. The variety of problems encountered is enormous, which is why it takes so long to become an expert. Probably 500 repairs are needed before one can feel really confident.

This account is based on my personal experience of over 600 operations conducted in Uganda (four hospitals), Sierra Leone (three hospitals), and the Addis Ababa Fistula Hospital in Ethiopia. I learnt a lot from a short visit to Dr Kees Waaldijk in Northern Nigeria, who has the largest personal experience in the world (13 000 cases).

Having helped many surgeons perform their first fistula operations, I can see the difficulties they have and understand the advice they need. Many of my operations have been performed in hospitals that have had no prior experience of fistula surgery, but this is no bar to success.

Naturally, fistula surgery is thought to be the province of gynaecologists and should rightly be part of their postgraduate training. In reality, many fistula surgeons have no formal gynaecological training and are simply good general surgeons who teach themselves following basic surgical principles.

One should not be discouraged by the fact of being able to operate on only some patients. A start has to be made somewhere, and one must not try to run before one can walk.

It is hard to imagine any operation that is more satisfying. It transforms the life of a young woman who would otherwise be an outcast.

Many surgeons have tried to tackle or have seen others attempt cases beyond their capability. Such cases usually fail, and everyone becomes discouraged. No surgeon likes failures. This text will show cases that should not be attempted, in order to avoid this embarrassment. Most African countries have hospitals where local experts operate or hospitals that are visited by outside experts. It is important to find out where they are and to refer all but the easy cases to them.

Once a surgeon has done a dozen or so easy fistula repairs, he or she may be encouraged to go further – but it is then important to try to obtain some training from an expert. Of all operations, fistula surgery is an example of one that cannot be learnt from reading a book (except the easy ones to be described here!). It is an art, and progress will be helped by a period of apprenticeship with someone more experienced. Several short visits are better than a single long one, in order to build up experience from one's own cases between visits. One of the problems of learning fistula surgery is that, working in a deep space, only the surgeon can really see what he or she is doing.

Once one understands the basic principles and the three-dimensional aspects of the pathology, to a large extent one has to work it out for oneself. To repair the bad cases, above average manual dexterity is required.

2 Understanding the Cause and Nature of Vesico-Vaginal Fistulae

Vesico-vaginal fistulae are caused simply by unrelieved obstructed labour. Prolonged pressure of the baby's head against the back of the pubic bone produces ischaemic necrosis of the intervening soft tissues, i.e. some part of the genital tract and bladder (Figure 1). In a labour taking long enough to produce this, the baby almost always dies. The head then softens and the mother eventually delivers a stillborn infant if she survives that long.

When the baby's head is stuck deep in the pelvis, the most common site for ischaemic injury is the urethro-vesical junction, as indicated in Figure 2, but other positions can occur either in isolation or confluently.

The extent of the injury depends on the duration of labour and the strength of the mother to survive this ordeal. In the most severe cases, ischaemia will affect the whole of the anterior wall of the vagina and sometimes the rectum as well, leading to a recto-vaginal fistula. Varying degrees of vaginal stenosis are common.

The prolonged pressure in the pelvis on the lumbar and sacral nerves may lead to neurological damage. In its most severe form, this causes complete paralysis of the lower limbs, but milder ischaemia will commonly cause foot drop. Fortunately, even those with a serious paralysis usually recover after many months, although foot drop will be the last to recover, if at all. The presence of neurological signs usually indicates a bad vesico-vaginal fistula.

The exact site, size and amount of scar are functions of the position of the baby's head when it gets stuck, and the duration of the obstruction.

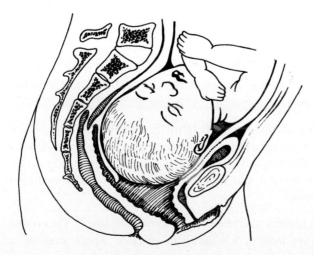

Figure 1 The area coloured blue is the first to undergo ischaemic necrosis.

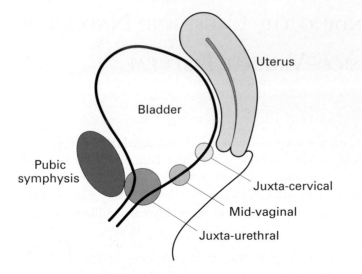

Figure 2 The various positions of ischaemic injury.

Many mothers die of exhaustion or a ruptured uterus in unrelieved obstruction – the fistula patients are the survivors.

Classification

A simple classification of vesico-vaginal fistulae is based on three factors:

- site
- size
- scar

The site of the fistula

Juxta-urethral (i.e. at the urethro-vesical junction) This is the commonest situation. Mild ischaemia will produce just a simple hole (Figure 3), but prolonged ischaemia will produce circumferential tissue loss where the urethra and bladder are separated to a variable extent (Figure 4).

Mid-vaginal Small defects 4 cm or more from the external urethral orifice are not that common, but are very easy to repair. Larger defects extend back as far as the cervix and laterally to the pubic bone.

Juxta-cervical (i.e. in the region of the cervix) (Figure 5) This is common where there is a high incidence of Caesarean section. Sometimes the defect extends into the cervical canal, with the anterior cervical canal being completely open (Figure 6). This presumably results from a vertical tear in the lower segment with associated bladder injury at Caesarean section.

Intra-cervical (i.e. between the bladder and the cervical canal) (Figure 7) This is not very common and almost always follows a Caesarean section. There may be a

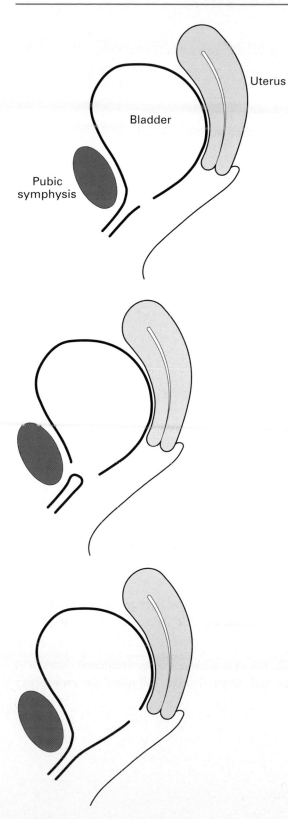

Figure 3 A simple juxta-urethral fistula.

Figure 4 A small circumferential juxta-urethral fistula. A gap exists between bladder and urethra. The latter is often blocked.

Figure 5 A juxta-cervical fistula.

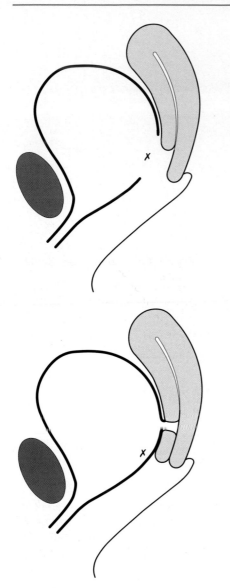

Figure 6 A large juxta-cervical fistula with an open anterior cervical canal (the cross indicates the ureteric orifice).

Figure 7 An intra-cervical fistula (the cross indicates the ureteric orifice).

history of a live baby, suggesting that the cause was iatrogenic. An alternative explanation is that the patient has been pushing for days with an incompletely dilated cervix.

Miscellaneous fistulae These include ureteric fistulae due to accidental damage at Caesarean section or hysterectomy, and vault fistulae following an emergency hysterectomy for a ruptured uterus.

The size of the fistula

Fistulae may be:

- tiny (admitting only a small probe)

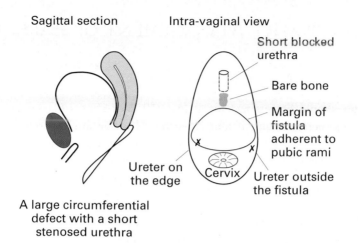

Figure 8 An extensive fistula. The whole of the anterior vaginal wall has been lost; there is a gap between the stenosed urethra and the anterior bladder wall. Bare bone is exposed at the back of the pubic symphysis. The antero-lateral margins of the bladder defect are adherent to the underside of the pubic arch, and the ureteric openings will be on the edge of or even outside the bladder, as indicated by the crosses on the intra-vaginal view.

- small (0.5–1.5 cm)

- medium (1.5–3 cm)

- large (>3 cm): these usually involve loss of most of the anterior vaginal wall and a circumferential loss of the urethro-vesical junction

- extensive (Figure 8)

The amount of scar

This varies from minimal when the margins of the fistula are soft and mobile to extreme scarring when the fistula margins are rigid and fixed. Scar also affects the lateral and posterior wall of the vagina, causing complete stenosis in extreme cases.

Scar is the big enemy, and any fistula with scar should be left to an experienced surgeon.

Prognosis

The critical factors are the length of the urethra and the amount of scar. Almost all defects can be closed (although bladder capacity may be reduced). However, if the urethra has been crushed, denervated and shortened, it will not function and the patient may have total stress incontinence. *The shorter the urethra and the greater the scar, the higher the chance of stress incontinence.* Destroyed urethras can be repaired, but the prognosis for continence is uncertain.

3 CONSERVATIVE MANAGEMENT OF EARLY CASES

The catheter should be retained for at least 10 days after a Caesarean section for prolonged obstructed labour. If there is urinary leakage after its removal, it should be reinserted immediately. Even on examination of the patient, the defect will probably not be visible because it will be out of sight in the region of the cervix. The patient should be kept on continuous drainage for at least 3–4 weeks. Many small fistulae will heal spontaneously if the bladder is kept empty.

After vaginal delivery, a leak of urine may indicate anything from a tiny hole to massive necrosis. The patient should be examined gently with a Sims speculum. If a large amount of slough is seen, it should be removed gently. This will probably reveal a large hole, and prolonged catheter drainage is unlikely to heal it. If a small defect is seen then 3–4 weeks' catheter drainage is essential. However, fistulae that have not healed spontaneously with drainage in 4 weeks are unlikely to do so.

Note that antibiotics have no part to play in the healing of fistulae – the cause is ischaemic necrosis, not infection.

Prevention at Caesarean section

In Uganda, two-thirds of patients with fistulae have had their obstructed labour relieved by Caesarean section – but too late. The remaining third have eventually delivered vaginally. In other countries, the incidence of Caesarean section may be different. For example, in Ethiopia, only 10% have had a Caesarean section because most people live in remote areas far from any hospital.

The ischaemic damage may have already occurred by the time of the Caesarean section, but the doctor can take steps to minimize any further damage. The lower segment will be very stretched and unhealthy. Remember that the bladder should always be dissected well down off the lower segment.

When the head is deeply impacted in the pelvis, it is better to get help to push up the head vaginally than to force a hand down between the head and the lower segment. This may produce vertical tears and increase the damage already done.

Tears in the lower segment can be difficult to suture, and sometime fistulae are produced when the doctor inadvertently picks up the bladder. This produces an intra-cervical fistula that can be quite a challenge to close and is not for the beginner.

How soon can the operation be performed?

Naturally, the sooner the patient can be cured the better. The longer she is incontinent of urine, the greater is the chance that she will be abandoned. This is almost inevitable when she perceives that there is no chance of cure.

Most surgeons advise waiting at least 3 months from the injury before operating. In the early months, the surrounding tissues are oedematous and hyperaemic, making them friable and difficult to handle. By 3 months, the surrounding tissues should be sufficiently mature. In spite of this, some surgeons have been very successful in closing selected fistulae before 3 months and have strongly recommended this approach. I recommend that the beginner follow traditional advice and delay repair for 3 months. After some experience has been gained, one can make exceptions to this rule.

4 Selection of Cases for the Beginner

Figures 9–13 show examples of the easier cases that are suitable for a beginner. Figures 14–18, on the other hand, show examples of more complex cases that should *not* be attempted by beginners.

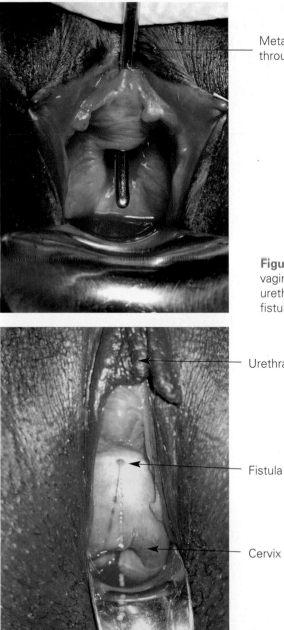

Metal catheter through the urethra

Figure 9 This is a medium vesico-vaginal fistula at the junction of the urethra and bladder. The margins of the fistula are soft and are clearly seen.

Urethra, hidden

Fistula

Cervix

Figure 10 This illustrates a tiny fistula of the mid-vagina. Urine can be seen leaking when the patient is asked to cough.

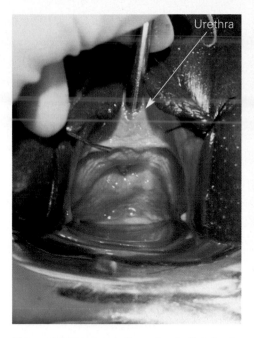

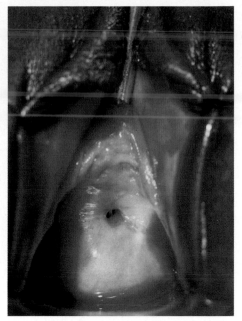

Figure 11 This is another simple fistula at the urethro-vesical junction. After a generous episiotomy, this will become much more accessible.

Figure 12 This is just about the easiest case one could hope to find. A metal catheter is in the urethra. The small fistula is just at the level of the urethro-vesical junction.

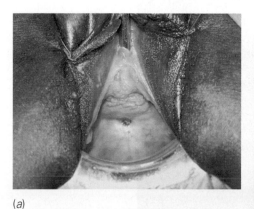

(a)

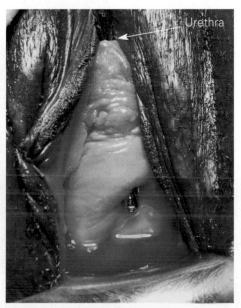

Figure 13 (a,b) Two more small mid-vaginal fistulae.

(b)

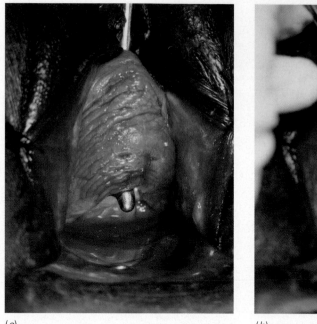

(a)

(b)

Figure 14 (*a,b*) This is a juxta-cervical fistula that extends high into an open cervical canal. It is a troublesome one to repair, but has an excellent prognosis because the urethro-vesical junction is normal.

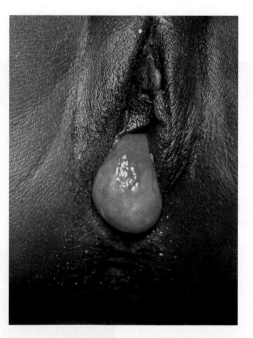

Figure 15 The defect in the vagina is so large that the bladder has prolapsed. This is perfectly curable by an expert surgeon.

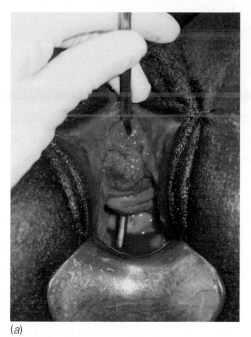
(a)

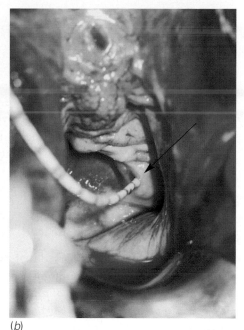
(b)

Figure 16 (*a,b*) This is a large fistula high in the vagina. When fully exposed after an episiotomy, the ureteric orifice is seen on the edge of the fistula (arrow). This would be quite easy for a regular fistula surgeon, but a novice could get into real difficulties.

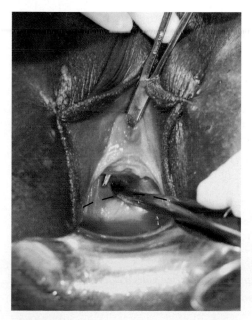

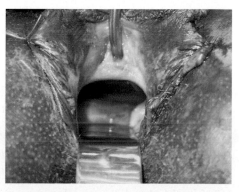

Figure 17 This looks like a small accessible fistula, but the vagina is almost completely stenosed beyond the fistula, as indicated by the forceps. Generous lateral incisions in the vaginal wall (indicated by the dashed line) are required to gain access to the fistula, which is otherwise quite an easy one to repair.

Figure 18 This massive defect was closed at the second attempt, but the patient had total urethral incontinence. A large rectal fistula (hidden here) was also present, but was cured (after a temporary colostomy).

13

5 Diagnosis

All of the photographs in Chapter 4 were taken in theatre before operation. This chapter deals with how one can recognize the type of fistula by history taking and examination. (Note that the data shown in *italics* in this chapter are taken from an analysis of over 500 consecutive fistula patients examined by the author in Uganda.)

History taking

The following details are required:

Symptoms It should be confirmed that the patient is wet all the time. If she is dry at night then she probably has not got a fistula. Ask if there is any leakage of faeces as well as urine. *(In Uganda, 6% of patients who delivered vaginally had a recto-vaginal as well as a vesico-vaginal fistula, but this combination was rarely seen if the patients had a Caesarean section. The incidence of recto-vaginal fistula in Ethiopia is much higher at around 15%; the reason for this difference is not known.)*

Age *(The mean age given was 26 years.)*

Parity *(50% were primiparous.)* If the patient is multiparous then which delivery caused the fistula? *(In 90%, it was the last pregnancy, but some women do become pregnant even with a fistula.)*

How long has the patient been wet? *(The mean duration of fistulae was 6 years range (1 month–36 years.)*

Mode of delivery Was childbirth by vaginal delivery or Caesarean? *(66% of fistula patients were delivered by Caesarean. The figure may be quite different in other countries. For instance, in Ethiopia, the figure is around 10%; in contrast to Uganda, most patients live in such remote areas that they have no chance of reaching a hospital at all.)*

Does the patient still menstruate? Amenorrhoea is not uncommon after such a traumatic childbirth, but if the patient had a Caesarean section then one should suspect a hysterectomy for a ruptured uterus. Some patients do not know that they have lost their uterus.

Did the child survive? *(In women developing a fistula after Caesarean section, 12% had a live baby. Only 4% of those delivering vaginally had a live baby.)*

Where did the delivery take place: home, maternity centre or hospital? *(About two-thirds of those delivering vaginally did so at home.)*

Have any attempts been made to repair the fistula? *(13% of patients presenting to the author with a fistula have had a previous unsuccessful attempt at repair. Patients sometimes hide this information for fear that they will be turned away.)*

Social history The majority of patients with a long-standing fistula are single and live a very restricted life. The longer they have had the fistula, the more likely they are to be alone.

Summary

History taking does not help that much in selecting the easy cases – a small hole leaks just as much as a big one. There are, however, some clues that should arouse suspicion of a bad injury:

- Neurological weakness (usually foot drop), even if it has recovered.

- Rectal fistulae *(6% after vaginal delivery, 1.6% after lower-segment Caesarean section in Uganda)* usually occur in association with a bad bladder injury. This does not apply to anal sphincter injuries, which often occur in isolation.

- Fistulae following a Caesarean section are often in the region of the cervix (due to a combination of ischaemia and operative trauma), but are sometimes just simple low vaginal fistulae.

- A fistula following hysterectomy for a ruptured uterus will usually be in the vault or be due to an accidental ureteric injury.

Examination

Inspection

1. Look for obvious urinary leak and urine dermatitis (Figure 19). (The dermatitis is caused by concentrated urine – ask the patient to drink more if it is not possible to operate immediately.)

2. Can the urethral orifice be seen? In very bad fistulae, it can be completely destroyed. *(2% in Uganda.)*

3. Is there any stenosis? (Figure 20).

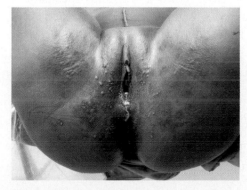

Figure 19 Urine dermatitis.

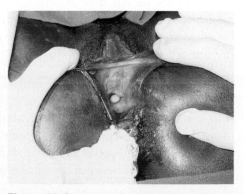

Figure 20 Severe vaginal stenosis seen on inspection.

Palpation by PV

Using the index finger gently:

1. Can any stenosis be felt? Smaller degrees are felt as a band of fibrous tissue around the lateral and posterior circumference at any depth in the vagina. In extreme cases, the whole of the vagina is stenosed.

2. Can a defect be felt in the anterior vaginal wall? This will range from a large defect where the finger immediately enters the bladder, to smaller defects that just admit the finger, to the smallest ones where no defect is felt at all. (With experience, one gets better at detecting the small ones.)

   – If a defect can be felt, where is it in relation to the urethra and the cervix?

   – If a fistula can be felt, consider the margins carefully. Are they soft and supple, a bit rigid or (in the worst cases) stuck to the pubic rami?

3. Can the cervix be identified? Does it feel normal? How deep is the vagina, has it been shortened?

The anterior cervix is often torn in fistula patients. Defects in this region are often difficult to feel unless they are large. When there has been a lot of tissue loss, the anterior vaginal wall is shortened and the cervix (or remnant) will be easily felt. If a small defect is felt that is not too close to the cervix and has soft margins with no vaginal stenosis then this is a suitable case for the beginner.

If preferred, the fistula can be inspected. This is best done with the patient in the lithotomy position, using a Sims speculum.

What should be done if the patient says she is wet but it is not possible to see any wetness or feel a fistula?

In this situation, the patient should be asked to drink plenty and then be re-examined (remember that many patients drink very little, especially if they know they are going to be examined). If it is thus confirmed that the patient is wet but a fistula cannot be felt then one should proceed as follows. If a Sims speculum is available, it should be used to expose the anterior vaginal wall. The patient should be asked to cough – a small fistula may be readily visible. The alternative is to perform a dye test as shown in Figure 21.

Ureteric fistulae

A ureter can be damaged accidentally during a Caesarean section, but injury is more likely during an emergency hysterectomy for a ruptured uterus. After the operation, urine leaks into the pelvis and some days later finds a way out through the lower segment incision or between the sutures in the vaginal vault.

To exclude a ureteric fistula, empty the bladder and insert a dry swab in the vagina. Ask the patient to drink and walk about. Re-examine after half an hour. If the swab

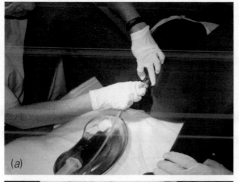

(a)

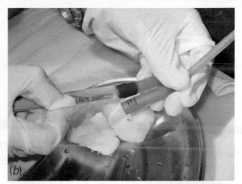

(b)

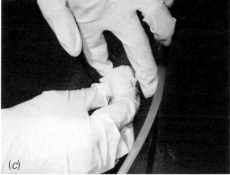

(c)

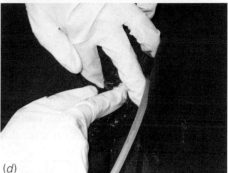

(d)

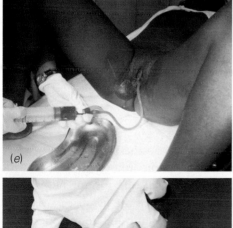

(e)

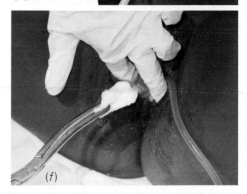

(f)

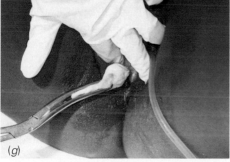

(g)

Figure 21 (*a,b*) Insert a catheter to perform a dye test. *Dilute* methylene blue (or gentian violet) is used. If it is too concentrated, it stains everything, resulting in difficulty in interpreting the test. Fill the balloon of the catheter and have two or three moist swabs ready to put in the vagina. (*c,d*) Put the swabs well into the vagina. (*e*) Slowly instil about 50 ml of dye. (*f,g*) Remove the swabs one by one. If the first is not stained but the second is stained blue, this confirms the presence of a fistula. If neither of the swabs is stained, there could still be a fistula, and the test should be repeated using up to 200 ml of dye. Wait for 20 minutes with the dye in the bladder. Sometimes the hole is very small, especially if it is between the cervix and the bladder. If this second test is negative, there may be an uretero-vaginal fistula.

is wet then a ureteric fistula is present. Although uncommon, it is very important to recognize because it can easily cured by an abdominal operation (see Chapter 10).

(21 ureteric fistulae were encountered in 520 wet patients in Uganda. In 9, the ureter had been injured at a Caesarean section, while in 12, the injury occurred during hysterectomy for a ruptured uterus. In 3 patients, there was a ureteric fistula coexisting with a simple vaginal fistula. These were not recognized until after the vesico-vaginal fistula had been repaired! They were easily cured by a second operation to implant the ureter into the bladder.)

Postpartum stress

This is occasionally troublesome and can be mistaken for a fistula. Take the catheter out, leaving the dye inside. Watch to see if it dribbles out of the urethra and then ask the patient to cough. If there is significant stress, dye will come out. The management is conservative with pelvic floor exercises. Another uncommon cause is the postpartum atonic bladder leading to overflow incontinence. This will settle after a period of continuous catheter drainage.

Rectal fistulae

Finally, do not forget to examine the posterior vaginal wall and anal sphincters. A rectal fistula with a simple fistula is highly unlikely, but an anal sphincter tear is not infrequent. If the patient is symptomatic, consider repair (see Chapter 11).

Selecting the easy cases by history taking and examination should now be possible

There is no need to perform an examination under anaesthesia in order to select cases. By all means examine the patient in the theatre in the lithotomy position with a good light and speculum without anaesthesia. If the fistula cannot be exposed without anaesthesia then it is not an easy case. Assuming that the fistula can easily be seen, it should be possible to go ahead and give the anaesthetic and do the operation. However, if a beginner has any doubts, they should not proceed – instead, wait for a really easy case.

Investigations

Haemoglobin above 10 g/100 ml is preferable, but a lower level can be accepted, as blood loss will be minimal for simple fistulae.

- Intravenous pyelography and ultrasound scan are not necessary, even for bad fistulae.

6 Preoperative Preparation

Explanation

Clearly, the patient must be prepared for what is going to happen in theatre and must give her consent. She must be informed about the length of postoperative stay, the duration the catheter will be kept in and the restrictions on her activities. Those who operate on difficult cases would be wise to warn the patient of the limitations of surgery to achieve a cure.

Bowel preparation

It is best to have the rectum empty during the operation in case there is any leakage though the anus. In ideal circumstances, the patient would have an enema the day before – but in reality, enemas are forgotten or given at the last minute, often leading to contamination during the operation. It is much better to give no enema at all and simply to be sure that the patient has been asked to open her bowels before coming to theatre. In the unusual event of troublesome anal leakage, I insert a temporary anal pursestring suture.

Hydration

Left to her own devices, the patient will come to theatre dehydrated, as she will be trying to reduce the amount of wetness. This is a bad thing for a number of reasons:

- She will be hypotensive under spinal anaesthesia.
- Dehydration increases the difficulty in identifying the ureteric orifices in those cases where this is necessary.

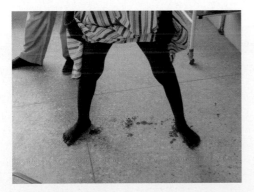

Figure 22 Preoperative hydration: if a patient has been drinking sufficiently, urine should drip when she stands with legs apart.

- Urine output will be poor after the operation, predisposing to catheter blockage. More intravenous fluids will be required during and after the operation.

Therefore, as soon as the decision has been made to operate, the patient should be asked to start drinking large volumes of any fluids, only stopping 4 hours before the operation. If she has been drinking sufficiently, urine should be seen dripping when she stands with her legs apart (Figure 22).

7 In Theatre

The anaesthetic

The choice of anaesthetic is not terribly important for simple cases and can be left to the preference of the anaesthetist. Spinal anaesthesia is used for most of my cases, but one anaesthetist prefers to work with ketamine alone, and this works well. The patient may, however, become restless during longer operations using ketamine.

Instruments

For simple fistulae, the following are all that are needed (Figure 23):

- Auvards speculum
- good-quality dissecting scissors
- toothed dissecting forceps
- Allis tissue forceps
- artery forceps
- metal catheter
- small probe
- No. 15 blade (not illustrated)

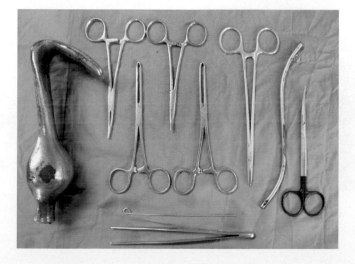

Figure 23 Instruments for simple fistula repair.

Sutures and needles (Figure 24)

Non-absorbable sutures should never be used, because a stone may form in the bladder much later.

The choice of suture may be determined by what is available. Plain catgut dissolves too fast but chromic catgut is fine. 2/0 or 3/0 Vicryl (or Dexon) would be the first choice of most surgeons, if available. For closure of the bladder, half-circle 25 mm round-bodied needles are best. For more advanced fistula work, eyed J needles are a great help. A larger cutting needle is used for suturing the vagina.

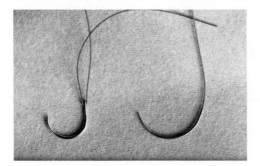

Figure 24 Needles for fistula repair: an eyed J needle mounted with 2/0 catgut and a swaged 25 mm half-circle needle with 2/0 Vicryl.

Operating table

An operating table that tilts and has shoulder rests (Figure 25) is essential for the full range of fistula surgery, but is *not* essential for simple fistulae.

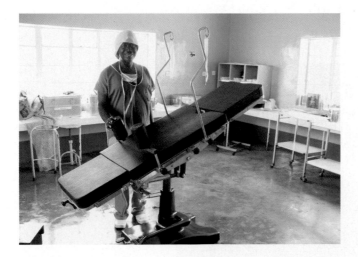

Figure 25 Tilting operating table with shoulder rests.

Lighting

A simple spotlight is sufficient (Figure 26). Note that poor lighting is not an excuse for not proceeding – one famous surgeon operates by daylight because the electricity supply is so erratic. If necessary, simply operate close to a large window (Figure 27).

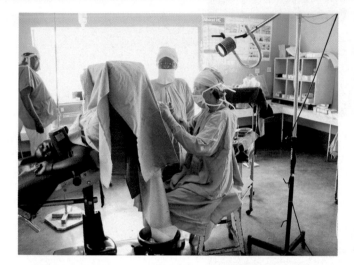

Figure 26 Operating spotlight.

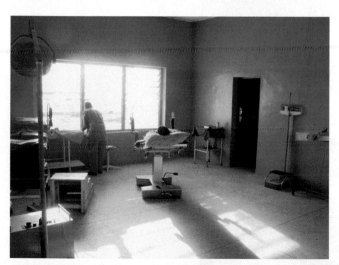

Figure 27 Operating by daylight.

Patient's position on the table

Even if the table will not tilt head down, make sure that the buttocks are well over the end of the table, the hips well flexed and the feet supported high out of the way (Figure 28).

23

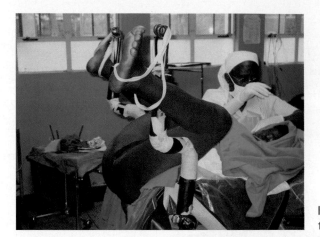

Figure 28 Patient positioned on the table.

Surgeon's position

Is the surgeon sitting comfortably (Figures 29 and 30)?

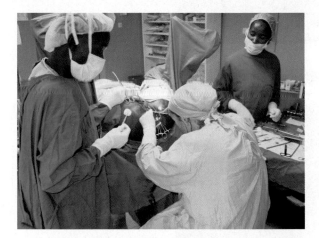

Figure 29 This surgeon is most uncomfortable: the table is too low.

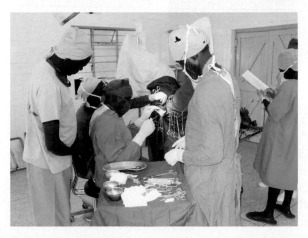

Figure 30 This is much better. Note the artery and Allis forceps clipped to the drapes.

8 A Simple Fistula Repair, Step By Step

The first step is to suture the labia to the thighs and cover the anus with a swab (Figure 31).

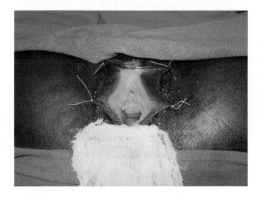

Figure 31 The labia are sutured to the thighs and the anus is covered with a swab.

Initial assessment (Figure 32)

- Record the site and size of the fistula.

- Estimate the distance from the external urethral orifice to the distal fistula margin.

- Estimate the distance from the proximal fistula margin to the cervix.

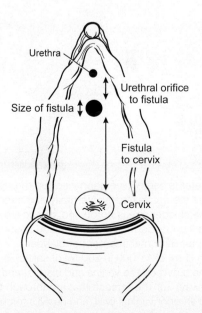

Urethra

Urethral orifice
to fistula

Size of fistula

Fistula
to cervix

Cervix

Figure 32 The measurements to be made.

An ideal beginner's case: an easy small soft fistula at the urethro-vesical junction (Figure 33a–t)

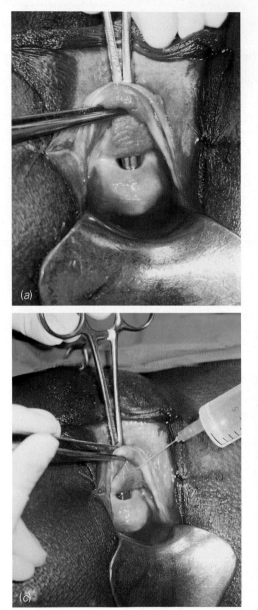

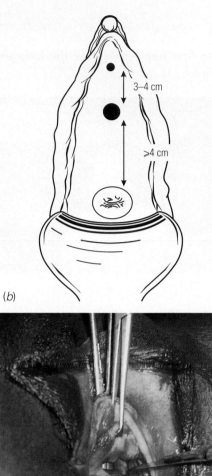

3–4 cm

>4 cm

(a)

(b)

(c)

(d)

Figure 33 (a,b) Artery forceps (usually a metal catheter is used) have been inserted through the urethra and held towards the operator to expose the fistula clearly. Normally, the interior of the bladder is explored with a metal catheter. The bladder size is noted and stones are felt for. Five percent of patients will have a stone in the bladder. The sensation and sound when tapping a stone is quite distinctive. (See Chapter 9 for management of bladder stones.) (c) Infiltration of a dilute adrenaline solution (1 ml of 1:1000 in 200 ml of saline) is optional. This may help in getting into the right plane between the vagina and bladder and will reduce bleeding (there should be very little anyway). (d) The forceps that are through the urethra are held towards the surgeon to steady the anterior vaginal wall, and an Allis forceps lifts up the mucosa over the urethra. The first incision is made on the posterior margin.

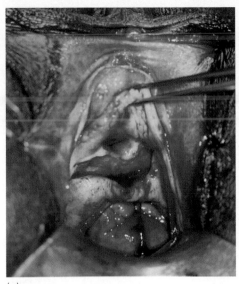

(e)

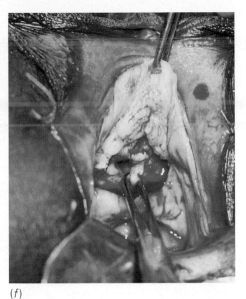

(f)

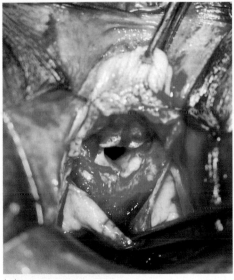

(g)

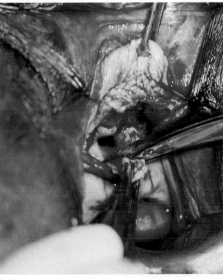

(h)

Figure 33 *(e)* The correct plane between bladder and vagina is identified. (*f*) The posterior dissection has been continued round to the sides to mobilize at least 1 cm beyond the fistula. The anterior incision has been commenced. It may help to make a little vertical extension towards the urethra. (*g*) The dissection is finished and the right and left antero-lateral flaps have been sutured to the labia well up out of the way. (*h*) Next, the vaginal mucosa at the fistula margin and any scar (very little in this case) is trimmed away.

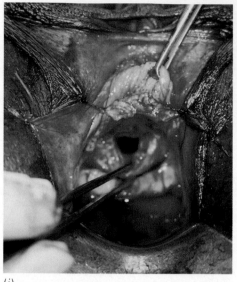
(i)

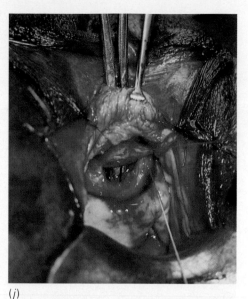
(j)

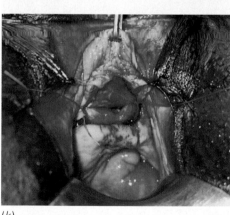
(k)

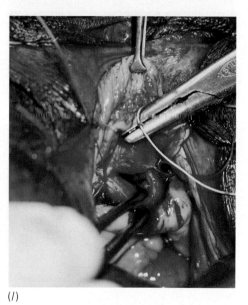
(l)

Figure 33 (i) The freshened margins of the fistula are now nicely exposed ready for suture. Start with the corners. (j) The first corner suture has been inserted beyond the margin of the fistula. (k) Both corner sutures have been inserted, tied and clipped. (l) Three more interrupted sutures, placed about 4 mm apart, will be required. Note that 'big bites' of bladder are taken, traversing the full thickness of the bladder wall but barely picking up the mucosa.

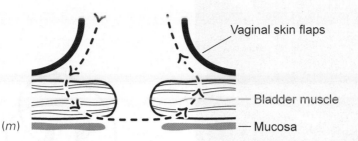

Vaginal skin flaps

Bladder muscle

Mucosa

(m)

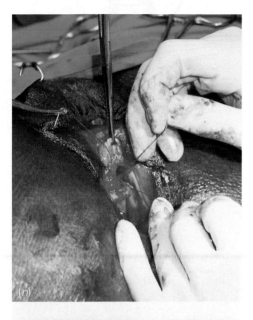

(n)

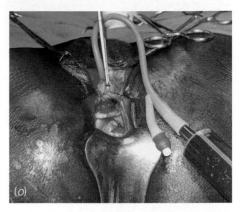

(o)

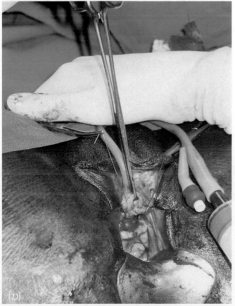

(p)

Figure 33 (*m*) Take good 'big bites' of bladder wall at least 0.5–1 cm from the edge. (*n*) The last suture is being tied. *Note*: never hold any instruments in the hands while tying knots since this makes it difficult to judge tension and tie accurately. (*o*) The repair has been completed in one layer. This is quite sufficient provided that 'big bites' have been taken and sutures have been placed accurately. A dye test should now be performed to check that the repair is watertight: use 60 ml of *dilute* methylene bluo (or gontian violet) introducod through a Foley catheter. (*p*) Press over the bladder or ask the patient to cough. In the unlikely event of a leak through the suture line, put in another suture. The main purpose of a dye test in a simple case is to exclude a second unsuspected fistula, especially an intra-cervical one if the patient has had a Caesarean section. This is rare but important to detect. It occurred in 4 out of the first 500 of my cases.

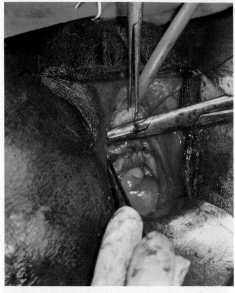

(q)

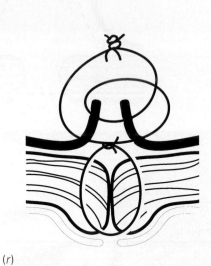

(r)

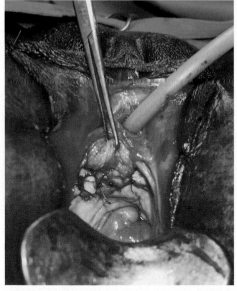

(s)

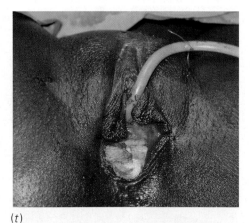

(t)

Figure 33 (q) Complete the vaginal closure with a layer of interrupted everting over-and-over mattress sutures. (r) Bladder and vaginal mucosa are sutured. (s) The repair is completed. (t) An antiseptic pack (in this case Betadine) is placed in the vagina. The catheter is sutured to the top of the labia.

9 PROBLEMS AND DIFFICULTIES

Difficult access

If access is difficult, the surgeon should not hesitate to perform an episiotomy, bilateral if necessary (Figure 34). These are easy to suture.

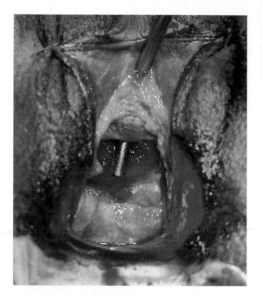

Figure 34 Bilateral episiotomies make access to this large fistula much better.

Blocked urethra

Sometimes a small fistula occurs at the urethro-vesical junction and the metal catheter will not pass through the proximal urethra due to a stricture. This indicates circumferential loss of tissue, even though the fistula appears small. Usually, gentle pressure will make the stricture give way. Then the fistula is repaired as described, remembering that it will be necessary to mobilize the fistula well beyond its lateral margins to release any scar.

This sort of fistula may be prone to develop a stricture some weeks after the repair, so it is important to insist on an early follow-up visit.

Bladder stones

These are uncommon, but can occur with small simple fistulae. It is essential to detect a stone at the start, as it should be removed and the repair postponed.

A metal catheter should always be used at the start, to sound out the bladder. The feel and sound on tapping a stone is quite distinctive. Sometimes a stone can be suspected during the examination, as this may be uncomfortable. The patient often has painful micturition and haematuria. The stone may be palpable bimanually.

Unless the stone is small or actually coming through the fistula (which is unusual), it should be removed by a separate generous suprapubic incision of the bladder (Figure 35). The bladder wall will be inflamed and thickened, and repair of the fistula should generally be delayed by at least 2 weeks.

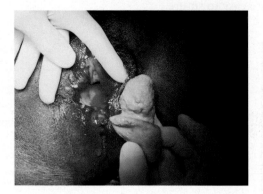

Figure 35 This stone was half in the bladder and half in the vagina, and was easily pulled out. Most stones are large and entirely intra-vesical, associated with a small fistula. Therefore suprapubic removal is recommended.

Ureteric involvement

The nearer the fistula is to the cervix, the greater the risk of ureteric involvement. Provided that the fistula is small and midline, the surgeon should not encounter the ureters. (See the discussion of juxta-cervical fistulae in Chapter 10.)

Duration of operation

The case described in Chapter 8 should take an experienced surgeon under 30 minutes. A beginner taking more than an hour either has problems with his or her technique or has selected the wrong sort of case.

10 Taking it Further

The beginner who feels confident having repaired some easy fistulae may feel able to progress to intermediate cases.

Scarred juxta-urethral fistulae

The essential step in repairing these is to get good exposure by making a generous episiotomy, bilateral if necessary (Figures 36 and 37). A tilting table really does make a difference to accessibility.

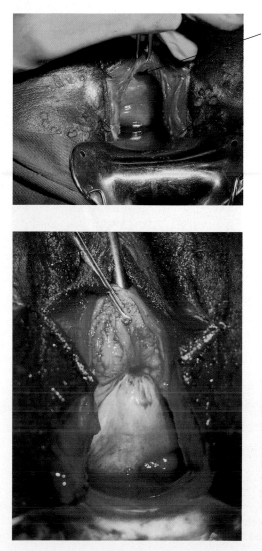

Fistula

Figure 36 In this case, the small fistula is only just visible because it is held up by scar tissue behind the pubic symphysis. An episiotomy and a tilting table will make access much easier.

Figure 37 This small juxta-urethral fistula was hidden behind the pubis. When the metal catheter is used to push the bladder base towards the surgeon and bilateral episiotomies are performed, the fistula becomes quite accessible.

The proximal urethra is often stenosed and the lateral margins may be adherent to the pubic rami.

The beginner should only tackle those cases that are lightly adherent until experience has been obtained. One should dissect laterally into the para-vesical space to completely free the margins of the fistula from bone. The lateral margins of the fistula must be freely mobilized before starting the repair, and there will be more scar to remove. This will make the defect larger than it was initially.

The distal margin of the fistula will be the proximal urethra, so great care should be taken to put the sutures in gently and accurately. Use a small needle but take good bites. If the sutures are cut out, this will make the repair much more difficult

Detached juxta-urethral fistulae

An apparently easy case of detached juxta-urethral fistula is shown in Figure 38(*a*); it has soft margins and is small.

When properly exposed, the urethra is seen to be detached from the bladder (Figure 38*b*). This is easy to re-anastomose after reflecting vaginal flaps. The anastomosis only needs to done round three-quarters of the circumference because there is continuity of muscle and mucosa on the deep aspect. This is an unusual case in being so mobile. Most detached urethras are adherent under the pubic arch (see Figure 4 in Chapter 2). The problem here is that the urethra is short (<2 cm), so there is a high risk of stress incontinence after repair.

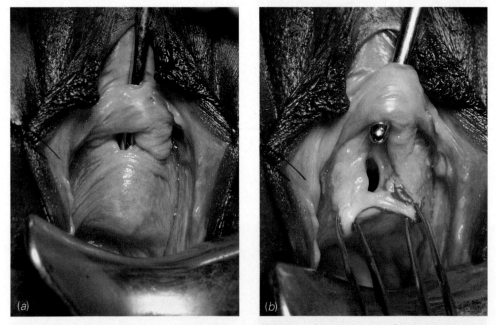

Figure 38 (*a*) This looks like an easy case – small with soft margins. (*b*) On proper exposure, the urethra is seen to be detached from the bladder.

The incidence of stress appears to be reduced by an ingenious little operation devised by Andrew Browning at the Addis Ababa Fistula Hospital (see the references in the Appendix). It consists of a sling under the urethro-vesical anastomosis using fibro-muscular tissue from the paravaginal tissue under the pubic arch. The vaginal skin is reflected more from the antero-lateral wall for exposure. A block of underlying fibromuscular tissue (part of the levator complex) is grasped with Allis forceps and a rectangular block of tissue is elevated (but remains attached

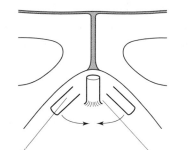

Fibromuscular
tissue from
paravaginal
tissue

Urethral
anastomosis

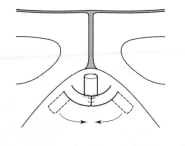

(a)

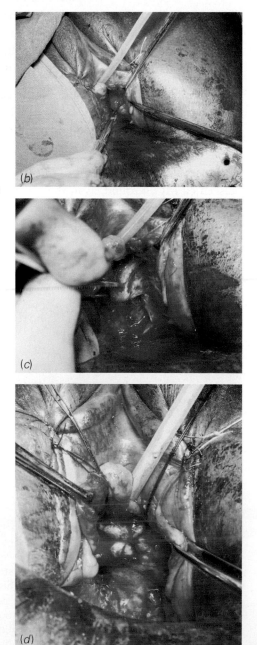

(b)

(c)

(d)

Figure 39 (a) The two strips of tissue are sutured together over the urethra. (b) Tissue is grasped from the lateral vaginal wall under the pubic ramus. (c) A block of fibromuscular tissue has been dissected out on the left-hand side. (d) The two blocks have been sutured together in the midline under the urethra. This produces the same effect as tension-free tape.

superiorly). The block of tissue is mobilized just enough to come to the midline to be sutured to one from the other side. It will come to lie just under the proximal urethra and urethro-vesical anastomosis. See Figure 39.

Smaller juxta-cervical fistulae

Two examples of smaller juxta-cervical fistulae are shown in Figure 40.

The accessibility of fistulae in the region of the cervix may depend on the parity of the patient. In the multiparous, the cervix will often come down, making access easy, as in the examples shown in Figure 40. In contrast, small juxta-cervical fistulae may be difficult to reach in primiparous patients, and are not for beginners.

In repairing fistulae in the region of the cervix, it is important to appreciate the risk to the ureteric orifices. The larger the fistula, the greater is the chance that these will be close to or at the fistula margin (Figures 41 and 42). As a rough guide, if a midline fistula is no more than 1 cm in diameter, the ureters will not be at risk.

Beginners should not attempt to repair a juxta-cervical fistula unless the margins can be seen clearly all round, as in the examples in Figure 40. If they cannot, the fistula may extend well up into the cervical canal and its repair may involve a difficult dissection. (See Figure 6 in Chapter 2 and Figure 14 in Chapter 4.)

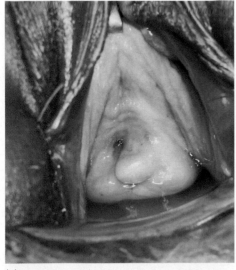
(a)

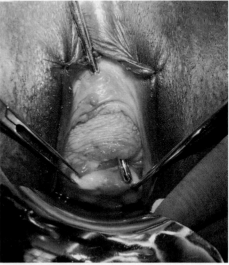
(b)

Figure 40 (a) This is a small juxta-cervical fistula where there is good access. It could be closed without identifying the ureters. (b) This is another example of a small simple juxta-cervical fistula. It is about 1 cm in diameter and 1 cm in front of the cervix. The urethra and bladder neck are undamaged, so the prognosis for continence will be excellent after repair. The ureteric orifices should be identified by the beginner in order to gain experience, although they should not be at risk in this small midline fistula.

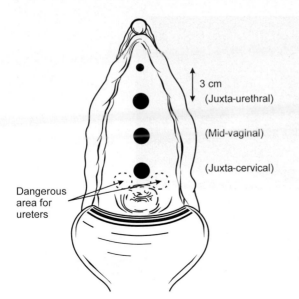

3 cm
(Juxta-urethral)

(Mid-vaginal)

(Juxta-cervical)

Dangerous
area for
ureters

Figure 41 Danger areas for
ureters.

The complete fistula surgeon must have access to ureteric catheters. Infant feeding tubes as an alternative are not very satisfactory as they are so soft. (In the author's series, repairing almost all fistulae at presentation, just over a quarter of cases were judged to need ureteric catheterization for identification and protection.) Ureteric catheters are not easy to find in Africa, so surgeons who are advancing to repair the larger mid-vaginal or juxta-cervical fistulae must learn to recognize the position of the orifices so as to avoid them in the repair.

The experienced surgeon can find them quickly by eye with a probe, but the best way when starting is to ask the anaesthetist to give 10 mg of furosemide intravenously. In 5 minutes, a brisk diuresis will make the orifices obvious if they are near the fistula margin. (This is another reason to make sure that the patient is well hydrated before arriving in theatre.) If the orifices are near the fistula margin and ureteric catheters are not available, they should be cannulated with a small metal probe. This can be held by an assistant during the mobilization and while the first inverting corner suture is inserted as illustrated in the case shown in Figure 43.

After repairing a fistula close to the cervix without using ureteric catheters, it is good practice to clamp the urethral catheter and to make quite sure that urine is produced. This is to exclude the very small chance that the ureteric orifices have been occluded in the repair.

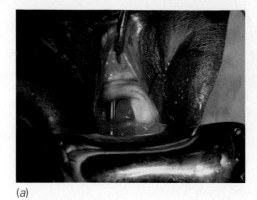

(a)

(b)

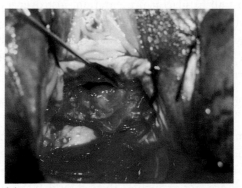

(c)

Figure 42 (*a*) This is a juxta-urethral fistula, but the cervix is close to the posterior margin under the Auvards speculum. This is caused by contraction of a large fistula. (*b*) A large fistula becomes smaller in the first 3 months. As the fistula contracts, the cervix is pulled down. So although the fistula appears to be small, it begins at the urethra and extends to the cervix. The ureters are at risk. (The cross indicates the position of the ureteric orifice.) (*c*) In this case, after mobilizing the vaginal flaps, a ureteric orifice has been found with a probe close to the left corner. The orifice should ideally be catheterized, but if no catheter were available then the corner suture could be inserted safely with the probe in place.

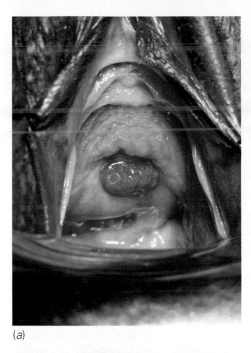

(a)

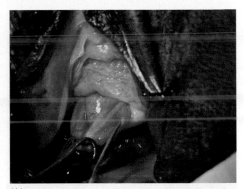

(b)

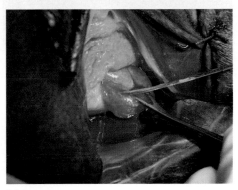

(c)

Figure 43 (a) A small juxta-cervical fistula. The left (b) and right (c) ureteric orifices have been identified close to the margin of the fistula with a probe. If ureteric catheters are not available, it is possible to close the fistula safely now they have been identified. (d) This fistula is 3 cm in diameter and the ureteric orifices are close to the edge of the fistula.

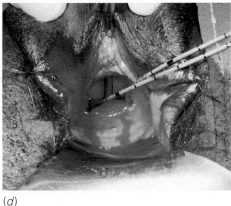

(d)

A simple juxta-cervical fistula (Figure 44)

The posterior margin of the fistula will be at the level of the cervix. It is best to start the operation by an anterior dissection between vagina and bladder. Make a vertical incision down the vaginal wall into the fistula margin. Enter the correct plane between the vagina and bladder through healthy tissue anteriorly. After working round the sides of the fistula, the antero-lateral flaps are sutured out of the way. This pulls the fistula up into view. Be sure to stay very close to the vaginal mucosa when dissecting laterally. If the bladder wall is entered, the ureter is at risk. The posterior margin is separated from the cervix. This is an easy plane to develop once any scar has been passed.

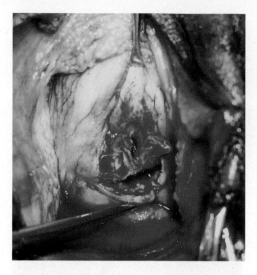

Figure 44 A small juxta-cervical fistula has been dissected from the cervix. The vagina has been separated from the bladder antero-laterally. Two sutures will close this fistula.

An easy intra-cervical fistula

Exceptionally, an intra-cervical fistula is very accessible, as in the case shown in Figure 45. It was easy to dissect between the bladder and cervix and close the fistula without identifying the ureteric orifices.

When is an abdominal repair appropriate?

Some fistula surgeons would say never. In practice, many surgeons starting fistula surgery will be experienced in abdominal but not vaginal surgery, so this approach is attractive – but beginners should beware.

It is essential to realize that any fistula that is below or likely to be close to the ureteric orifices should *not be attempted from above*. An experienced urologist may be able to do this, but it needs full abdominal relaxation, proper retractors, good light and an ability to catheterize the ureters from inside the bladder.

There are only three situations where a fistula can be repaired quite easily from above. For the novice fistula surgeon, this may be the best option – provided that the case is carefully selected.

The vault fistula after emergency hysterectomy for a ruptured uterus

Most of these are perfectly accessible from the vagina provided that they will come down, but an abdominal repair is an option for the inexperienced vaginal surgeon.

Careful bimanual examination will give an indication as to how close the fistula will come to the anterior abdominal wall. If it comes sufficiently close then this will be a good case to do from above, provided, of course, that there is good lighting and a good selection of instruments and deep retractors.

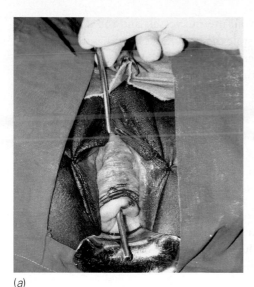

(a)

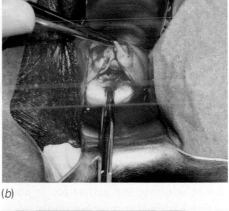

(b)

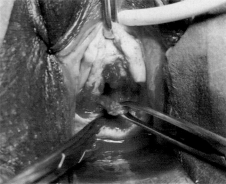

(c)

Figure 45 (a) An easily accessible intra-cervical fistula. (b) The space between the bladder and cervix has been developed. (c) The defect in the bladder can now be seen and is ready for suture.

The bladder should be exposed and mobilized from above and opened in the midline to inspect the interior. The fistula should be visible. The bladder incision is continued down to the fistula, and the bladder is separated from the vagina before each is closed in one layer. If the fistula is lower than expected then the ureteric orifices should be identified, if necessary with the help of furosemide. If the case has been selected wisely, the fistula should be well above the ureteric openings.

The post-Caesarean intra-cervical fistula

The regular fistula surgeon will learn to repair these from below by dissecting up between the cervix and bladder.

There is just one situation where the repair can be quite easy from above, namely following an iatrogenic injury without any ischaemic component. This can be suspected when the patient gives the story that she was delivered of a live baby, and yet is shown to have a leak through the cervix. The fistula is almost always caused by accidental suture of the bladder into the lower uterine segment. In this case, repair is quite possible from above by dissecting between the uterus, cervix and bladder. The hole is often tiny. Stay in the midline to avoid uterine vessels and the ureters, and if the fistula does not come into view easily, split the bladder vertically until the fistula is reached. It should be above the ureteric orifices: if there is any doubt, give furosemide to identify and avoid them. A tiny hole in the cervix does not need to be closed.

If the delivery by Caesarean section was a stillbirth, an abdominal repair should not be attempted, even if vaginal examination suggests that the fistula is intra-cervical. Labour long enough to cause death of the baby will produce an ischaemic injury. The fistula may turn out to be larger and lower than expected and will be very difficult and unsafe to access from above (except for experienced urologists).

Before selecting any patient for an abdominal repair, make absolutely certain by dye test and vaginal inspection under anaesthesia that the leak is coming through the cervix and not through an occult hole in the vagina (except, of course, for the post-hysterectomy vault fistula, in which case a final decision on approach can be made).

The ureteric fistula

If a ureteric injury occurs after a Caesarean section or hysterectomy, it will be deep in the pelvis. If the ureter is dissected and divided just above the level of injury, it will reach the bladder. In my 21 cases, it has not been necessary to perform any bladder-lengthening manoeuvres such as the Boari flap or psoas hitch stitch. The dome of the bladder is opened and the ureter is drawn into the bladder through a separate stab incision. See Figure 46.

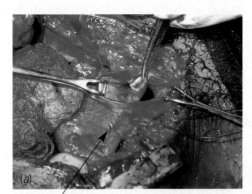

Ureter through
bladder wall

Anastomosis
inside bladder

Figure 46 (*a*) The ureter has been mobilized and drawn into the opened bladder. (*b*) The ureter has been sutured to the bladder mucosa and will be additionally secured by sutures placed in the outer bladder wall.

Which side?

The injured ureter is almost always dilated and scar tissue can be felt at the site of injury. Occasionally, it can be difficult to decide by inspection and palpation alone which ureter is damaged. In this situation, open the bladder through the fundus and look inside. Give furosemide, and expose the ureteric orifices with a retractor and confirm that one ureter is connected to the bladder and the other is not.

Labial fat grafts and fistula repair

At the Addis Ababa Fistula Hospital, fat grafts are used for all but simple repairs. It is believed that this increases the success rate, especially for the complex cases (although there is no proof of this). However, there are some experienced fistula surgeons who rarely use fat grafts – without apparently compromising their results. I believe that there is a place for fat grafts (especially following a difficult repair) but my own use has fallen to less than 10% of all cases. All are agreed that simple fistulae do not need a fat graft, so this procedure is not described in this account for novice fistula surgeons.

Antibiotics

Some surgeons give no antibiotics, while others prescribe them throughout the postoperative period. It is well known that infection usually results from contamination during the operation, so it is my practice to give a single intravenous dose of gentamicin 160 mg at the start of surgery. I would only continue with antibiotics for 24 hours if there had been accidental faecal contamination of a repair or if there had been a sphincter repair as well. My choice would be gentamicin 80 mg and metronidazole 500 mg intravenously 8 hourly.

11 Repair of Anal Sphincter Injuries

Immediate repair

Tears seen within 24 hours of delivery should be repaired at once. This is not a minor operation. The patient's future continence depends on the skill of the repair.

This must be done in a theatre with good lighting, instruments and assistance. Repair under local anaesthesia is possible, but it might be better to have the patient under spinal or general anaesthesia.

It is important to realize that the torn anal sphincters retract to the 3 and 9 o 'clock positions. Close the ano-rectal mucosa first, then identify the torn ends of the external sphincter (the internal sphincter cannot be identified as a separate layer). Suture these accurately, taking quite big 'bites', using Vicryl if possible. Three to four sutures will be needed. Then close the vagina and perineal skin using good mattress sutures to build up the perineal body.

Secondary repair

If the repair cannot be done immediately, it is best to wait several weeks. Sometimes patients with an old complete tear say they have no symptoms, so it is important to be sure that the patient really does have troublesome faecal leakage before recommending repair. In the best hands, only 80% of repairs restore complete continence.

Again it is important to realize that the torn ends of the sphincter have retracted round half the anal circumference, and simply freshening and suturing the margins of the tear is unlikely to give a good result.

Procedure

The procedure for repair of an anal sphincter tear is shown in Figure 47.

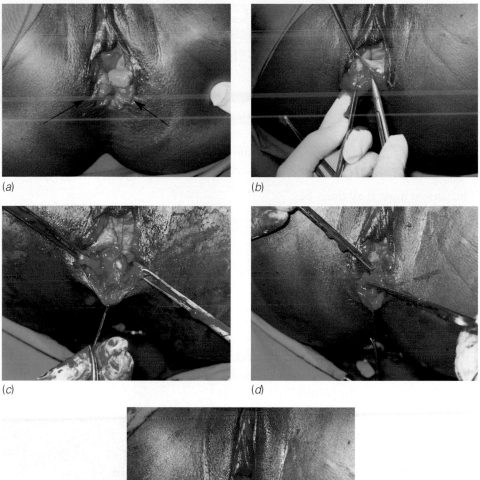

(a)

(b)

(c)

(d)

(e)

Figure 47 (*a*) A late complete anal sphincter tear. The arrows indicate the position of the retracted sphincter ends. (*b*) The vaginal mucosa is separated from the ano-rectal mucosa and then the ends of the sphincter are identified postero-laterally. Aim to mobilize a block of tissue that contains the sphincter end. If only muscle is mobilized, it will easily tear. (*c*) The ano-rectal mucosa has been repaired, and blocks of tissue containing the external sphincter are held in forceps. (*d*) Aim to repair the sphincters by overlapping the two blocks of tissue. The mobilized tissue should contain some scar tissue around the sphincter. Pure sphincter muscle would not hold sutures well. (*e*) The completed repair. The initial transverse incision has been converted to a vertical one. There is tension in the middle of the suture line, so the wound has been left open here. Should infection or bleeding occur, the repair would not be compromised.

12 POSTOPERATIVE CARE OF THE FISTULA PATIENT

A good operation can be ruined by neglectful aftercare. It is the surgeon's responsibility to ensure that the nurses and carers know what is required. In reality, nurses will be in short supply and may not have seen a fistula repair before.

The patient must at all times be:

- draining
- drinking
- dry

Drainage

Free drainage of urine at all times depends on adequate catheter care. If a catheter blocks, urine may pass alongside it or, much worse, find a way through the repair. Then the scene is set for failure.

Principles of catheter care

- Nothing must pull on the catheter.
- The catheter must not become blocked or fall out.

The catheter is secured in theatre with a suture to the labia. This prevents accidental traction on the catheter as the patient is moved from the theatre to the ward and at other times. The catheter may additionally be strapped to the thigh to prevent discomfort due to the labial suture (Figure 48). However, strapping alone is not enough – it easily comes off.

Drainage bags or not?

Closed drainage is ideal if the nursing care is excellent and good-quality bags

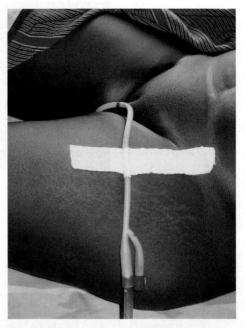

Figure 48 Strapping to the thigh is acceptable to prevent discomfort from the suture through the labia.

are available (Figure 49*a*). However, these conditions are not often met in Africa. In addition, a number of problems may arise when drainage bags are used (Figure 49*b*,*c*), although some can be circumvented (Figure 49*d*) and a bag can have advantages (Figure 49*e*).

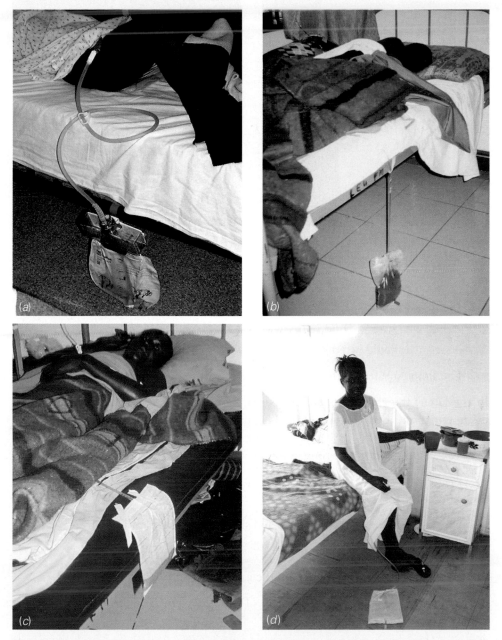

Figure 49 (*a*) This high-quality system is ideal, but is expensive and would rarely be available in an African setting. (*b*) This bag has already become full and if further neglected will overfill and pull loose from the bed, pulling the catheter out of the patient. (*c*) This bag will soon fall off the bed and pull on the catheter. (*d*) With long tubing, the bag can lie on the floor.

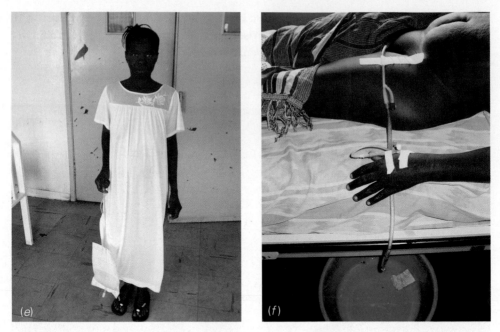

Figure 49 (*e*) A good-quality drainable bag does make ambulant care easy. (*f*) Open drainage

In general, however:

- Unless there is no doubt that staff can look after a drainable bag, a simple alternative should be employed.

- The simplest safest option is open catheter drainage.

In the latter, the catheter is connected to plastic tubing and drains directly into a basin under the bed (Figure 49*f*). The patient can move freely in the bed and nothing will pull on her catheter. It is easy to see that urine is draining by watching the drips, and little can go wrong at night.

Blocked catheter

This is an emergency! The symptoms and signs of a blocked catheter are:

- The patient feels a full bladder.

- She is wet (due to leakage around the catheter or through the repair).

- Urine stops dripping into the basin. This would not be noticed for some time when closed drainage is used.

Action must be taken immediately:

- Examine the catheter – it may be twisted or blocked (Figure 50). The remedy is to change the tubing and make the patient drink more.

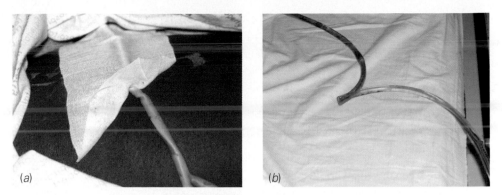

Figure 50 (*a*) A twisted catheter. (*b*) A kinked catheter. Note that the urine is concentrated and contains cloudy deposits.

- Examine the patient. Is the bladder palpable? If so, unblock the catheter at once by gentle irrigation with a bladder syringe. If this does not work, change the catheter. If there is any doubt about drainage, always irrigate the catheter.

Drinking

A high fluid intake is essential. This should start before operation and continue until after removal of the catheter. This means at least 4–5 litres a day. Many patients may be reluctant to drink. They have been accustomed to drinking little to reduce their wetness. They may be afraid that drinking too much will spoil the repair. Reassure them.

Concentrated urine predisposes to urinary infection and to accumulation of debris, which predisposes to blockage.

There is no need to record urine output except for the immediate postoperative period. With the open drainage method, it is easy to see at a glance whether the patient is drinking enough (Figures 51 and 52) – look for the drips and look at the colour.

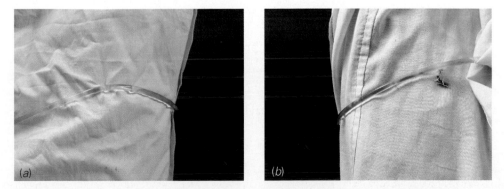

Figure 51 (*a*) The urine should be like water. (*b*) This urine is too concentrated.

Dryness

The patient must be dry. Possible causes of wetness are:

- A blocked catheter: this is serious but easily remedied. It should be uncommon if the patient has a high fluid intake.

- A failed repair: this should be very unlikely if the surgeon has selected an easy case and repaired it well. If there is any doubt, a dye test should be performed.

- Urethral leakage: as well as draining via the catheter, urine will sometimes leak alongside it, which may suggest that the urethra has poor function. Careful inspection of the urethra while performing bladder irrigation will identify this problem.

- A second fistula has been missed: a simple low vesico-vaginal fistula may coexist with an intra-cervical or a ureteric fistula (both could be iatrogenic at the time of a Caesarean section or hysterectomy for a ruptured uterus). Note that a dye test at the end of the repair should reveal the uterine fistula (unless it is tiny), but would not show a ureteric leak.

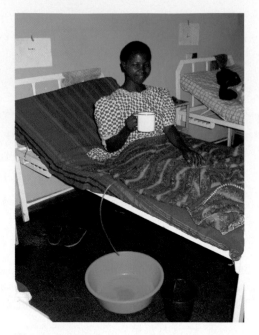

Figure 52 Make sure that the patient has a plentiful supply of water and look for the urine dripping into the basin.

A simple record of the patient's operation and a postoperative care plan should be kept on the foot of the bed or on the wall where it can be easily seen by all (Figure 53).

Other aspects of postoperative care

Perineal toilet

Twice daily vulval washing is essential, paying particular attention to the catheter as it comes out of the urethra.

Vaginal packing

This should be removed on day 2 (the day of operation is day 0).

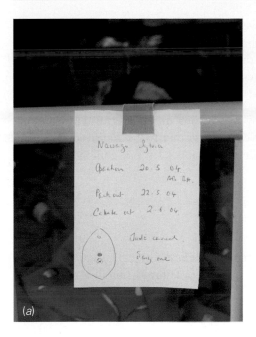

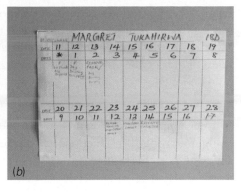

(b)

(a)

Figure 53 (a) A record can be kept on the end of the bed. (b) Alternatively, a record can be fixed to the wall.

Mobilization

The patient is allowed out of bed after removal of the vaginal pack. If she has open drainage, she can use a bucket to collect urine and can carry this around with her (Figure 54). This works perfectly well, but remember to keep the patient drinking lots of fluid.

Removal of the catheter

Many surgeons leave the catheter in for 14 days after all fistula repairs, but for simple ones 12 days are sufficient.

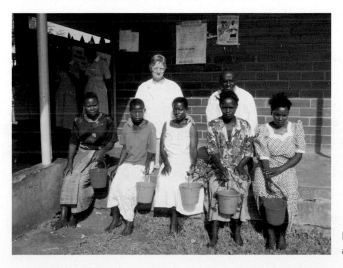

Figure 54 Patients up and about with their buckets.

Just before the catheter is due to be removed, it is advisable to perform a simple dye test on the ward or in theatre. Provided that there is no leakage, simply remove the catheter in the morning and encourage the patient to pass urine at least every 2 hours. Later, as her bladder becomes accustomed to distension, she will be able to hold on longer.

Some people advocate bladder training, by which they mean intermittent clamping and unclamping for 48 hours before the catheter is due to be removed. This can easily go wrong if instructions are misunderstood, and I am not convinced there is any benefit in this regime.

Has the repair failed?

A leak requires a dye test unless gentle irrigation demonstrates leakage around the catheter. A leak from the vagina on dye test indicates a failure – but all is not lost.

Early leak – in the first week

This is bad news, and usually means that the repair has failed. It should be rare after the easy repairs described here, but will be more of a problem as the difficult ones are tackled. If more urine is draining through the catheter than the vagina, it is worth keeping the catheter as long as this is the case in the small hope that healing might occur.

Late leak – in the second week or later

Occasionally, even simple repairs develop a leak during the second week. This may be a secondary breakdown due to infection. In these cases, as the fistula margins are not under tension and have a good blood supply, there is every chance that the defect will close with prolonged bladder drainage. Keep the catheter in for up to 3–4 weeks in total as long as the leak is diminishing.

The later the leak, the better the prognosis

It may help to keep the patient in bed lying and sleeping face down (Figure 55). In this position, the hole in the base of the bladder will be uppermost and the catheter tip will be below it (i.e. sump drainage).

One of my patients was discharged home dry after 14 days, but returned wet for my next visit 6 months later.

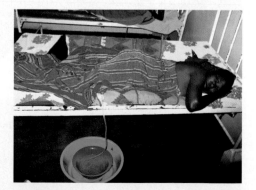

Figure 55 Nurse the patient prone if she has a secondary breakdown.

She said she had become wet the day she arrived home and attributed this to the long walk. If only she had returned and had a further period of catheter drainage, the secondary breakdown would almost certainly have healed.

It is a good idea for patients to stay for a few days after removal of the catheter, especially if they have come far.

Predischarge advice

Abstinence from sexual relationships for 3 months

Occasionally, we see patients who went home dry but report a leak developing after a few weeks. Perhaps they were not able to abstain.

Caesarean section for all future pregnancies

Do not forget to discuss family planning issues, including tubal ligation where relevant. Future pregnancies must be delivered by Caesarean section. If the obstructed labour was due to a malpresentation, the patient could in theory deliver vaginally in future, but as skilled obstetric care is rarely available, it is best to insist on a Caesarean section for all subsequent deliveries. From time to time, we do see patients with a recurrent fistula because they have not been able to get to hospital for this.

Return for follow-up consultation

It is so important for surgeons to know their results that patients should be given financial help to return. One can only really know one's results if the patient returns for a follow-up visit. Make sure that you see the patients yourself if possible.

Possible late problems

Urinary infections

These should be uncommon, provided that a high urine output is maintained. A late postoperative infection could be caused by a stricture with retention or by a missed bladder stone. Where limited laboratory facilities exist, inspection of the urine should be enough to make the diagnosis.

Stress incontinence

A little leakage for the first few days after catheter removal is quite common, but permanent stress incontinence should be rare after repair of a simple fistula unless the urethra was short.

Stress incontinence is unfortunately common after repair of complex fistulae where there has been significant destruction of the urethra and loss of bladder volume.

Pelvic floor exercises may help, but only if there has been minimal destruction of the normal continence mechanism. There are a number of surgical options for treatment of stress incontinence after fistula surgery, with only a modest success rate.

Stricture

Any patient who had a stricture of the proximal urethra at the time of repair is at risk of postoperative stenosis. Any urinary symptoms require examination of the urethra with dilators. Small Hegar dilators are ideal for this. Small strictures should yield readily to dilatation. Regular dilatation will prevent the stricture from becoming resistant.

Sexual difficulties

In spite of a good repair without any vaginal stenosis, some women are reluctant to resume sexual relations. There may be a number of reasons for this, and sensitive enquiry and examination are required to reassure these patients.

Audit your work

Surgeons should keep an accurate record and notes of all of their cases. These cases may be infrequent at first, so keeping good records is essential to build up experience.

13 Comparison of Two Approaches to Fistula Repair

It is important to realize that there are many routes to successful repair as long as basic principles and common sense are followed. As an example of the diverse approaches that can be used, I have contrasted the methods followed by the two most experienced centres in the world. They are quite different, but they both achieve excellent results.

	Addis Ababa, Ethiopia (Dr Hamlin)	Katsina, Nigeria (Dr Waaldijk)
Preoperative preparation		
Preoperative drinking	Not emphasized	Strongly emphasized
Preoperative enemas	Given for 2 days	Not given
Operative details		
IV fluids	24 hours	Rarely used
Antibiotics	10 days[a]	None
Episiotomy	Infrequent	Large and liberal use
Extent of dissection	Extensive	Minimal
Layers	2	1
Fat graft	Often	Rarely
Postoperative care		
Catheter drainage	Open, into a kidney dish in bed	Open, into a bucket
Ureteric catheters	Retained for 1 week	Removed at the end of the operation in most cases
Bed rest	2 weeks	2 days

[a]Controlled clinical trial now in progress.

Appendix: Books, Articles and Videos

Books

Moir C. *The Vesico-Vaginal Fistula*.

This classic monograph, first published in 1961, is an excellent introduction to fistula surgery but is now out of print. A limited reprint has been made for the Addis Ababa Fistula Hospital, and may be obtained from the hospital at Box 3609, Addis Ababa, Ethiopia.

Waaldijk K. *Step by Step Surgery of Vesico Vaginal Fistulas*. This was published in 1994 and is obtainable from Teaching Aids At Low Cost (TALC), Box 49, St Albans, Herts AL1 5TX, UK (info@talcuk.org).

This is essential reading for any serious fistula surgeon. It is based on Kees Waaldijk's personal experience, which is the largest in the world. It is very detailed and well illustrated, but the beginner might find some parts hard to follow. Some sections are in need of updating in view of Dr Waaldijk's evolving experience.

Goh J, Krause H. *Female Genital Tract Fistula*. Herston, Queensland: University of Queensland Press, 2004 (obtainable from the Medical Bookshop, University of Queensland, Herston Road, Herston, Queensland 4006, Australia; medicalbookshop@uq.net.au).

This is a very useful, well-illustrated and practical account of the whole range of obstetric and gynaecological fistulae.

Zacharin RF. *Obstetric Fistula*. New York: Springer-Verlag, 1987.

This is a comprehensive and very interesting account of the historical aspects of fistula repair, but would be of little help to the beginner. It contains a chapter about the early days of the Addis Ababa Fistula Hospital.

Hamlin C. *The Hospital by the River*. Macmillan Australia, 2001/Oxford: Monarch Books, 2004.

This is a fascinating account of Catherine Hamlin's dedicated work at the Addis Ababa Fistula Hospital.

WHO Manual for the Care of VVF Patients. In preparation. This will contain chapters on social integration and rehabilitation, nursing care, physiotherapy and operative principles. WHO Publications, 20 Avenue Appia, 1211 Geneva 27, Switzerland (bookorder@who.int).

Articles

Arrowsmith S, Hamlin EC, Wall LL. Obstructed labor injury complex: obstetric fistula formation and the multifaceted morbidity of maternal birth trauma in the developing world. CME review article. *Obstet Gynaecol Surg* 1996; **51**: 568–74.

Browning A. Prevention of residual urinary incontinence following successful repair of obstetric vesico-vaginal fistula using a fibro-muscular sling. *BJOG* 2004; **111**: 357–61.

Hamlin EC, Muleta M, Kennedy R. Providing an obstetric fistula service. *Br J Urol Int* 2000; **89**: 50–3.

Kelly J. Urogynaecology in the developing world. In: *Clinical Urogynaecology* (Stanton J, Monga A, eds). Edinburgh: Churchill Livingstone, 2000.

Kelly J. Repair of obstetric fistulae. *Obstet Gynaecol* 2002; **4**: 205–11.

Kelly J, Kwast BE. Epidemiological study of vesico-vaginal fistula in Ethiopia. *Int Urogynaecol J* 1993; **4**: 278–81.

Teaching videos (PAL system)

- *Repair of Simple Vesico-Vaginal Fistula by Catherine Hamlin* (40 minutes)

- *More Repairs from the Addis Ababa Fistula Hospital* (40 minutes)

It is planned to make these available in DVD format. They are obtainable from Brian Hancock, 21 Yealand Road, Yealand Conyers, Lancashire LA5 9SG, UK (brian@yealand.demon.co.uk).

ACKNOWLEDGEMENTS

Many people have helped and inspired me to take up fistula surgery – especially the staff of the Addis Ababa Fistula Hospital, but I should also like to thank Dr John Kelly, Dr Moira Lynch, Dr Tom Raassen and Dr Andrew Browning.

I would like to dedicate this small publication to Dr Catherine Hamlin and the staff of the Addis Ababa Fistula Hospital (Figure 56) – especially to Mamitu Gashe, the patient turned surgeon. Her skill is legendary, and she assisted and guided me at many of my early repairs as she has done for so many surgeons who come to learn at the Addis Ababa Fistula Hospital.

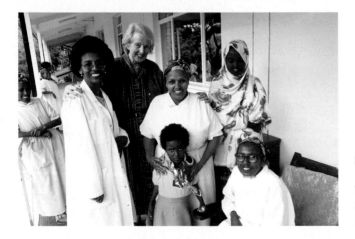

Figure 56 Dr Catherine Hamlin with Dr Ambye Woldemichael on her right and Mamitu Gashe on her left.

I would also like to acknowledge the teaching and example of Dr Kees Waaldijk in Northern Nigeria, who has done so much to demonstrate how fistula surgery can be performed with the bare minimum of facilities (Figure 57).

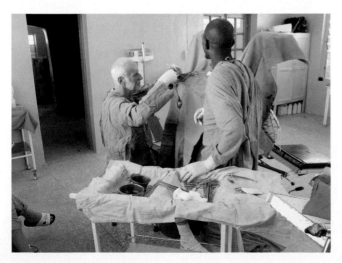

Figure 57 Dr Kees Waaldijk operating in Katsina, Northern Nigeria.

Finally, I am most grateful to the following hospitals that have so willingly allowed me to operate and take photographs for use in this publication.

- Uganda: Kamuli Mission Hospital, Busoga District; Kitovu Mission Hospital, Masaka District; Nsambya Mission Hospital, Kampala; Lira Government Hospital, Northern Uganda.

- Nigeria: Katsina Hospital.

- Ethiopia: The Addis Ababa Fistula Hospital.

- Sierra Leone: Kambia District Government Hospital; Princess Christian Maternity Hospital Freetown.

- Mercy ships: in Gambia, Sierra Leone and Benin (mercyships.org).

INDEX

A
abdominal surgery 40–2
    indications and contraindications 40
    post-Caesarean intra-cervical fistulae
        41–2
    selection of patients for repair 42
    ureteric fistulae 42
    vault fistulae 40–1
Addis Ababa methods, *vs* Katsina methods
    55
anaesthetic 21
anal sphincter injury repairs 44–5
    immediate *vs* secondary 44
antibiotic cover 43
approaches to fistula repair compared 55
audit 54

B
bladder, prolapse 12
bladder stones 31–2
'bladder training', contraindications 52
blocked urethra 31
books, articles and videos 56–7

C
Caesarean section, prevention of fistulae
    8–9
classification 4
    beginner cases 10–12
    complex cases 12–13
    danger areas for ureters 37
comparison of approaches to fistula repair
    55
conservative management, early cases 8–9

D
diagnosis 14–18
    history-taking 14–15
    inspection 15–18
    investigations 18
    palpation 16
    post-partum stress 18

rectal fistulae 18
ureteric fistulae 16–18
discharge, pre-discharge advice 53
drinking, postoperative care 49
dye test 17, 29

E
episiotomies 31
extensive fistulae 7, 12–13
    see also classification

F
fat grafts for fistula repair 43
fibromuscular urethro-vesical sling,
    prevention of stress incontinence
    35–6
fistula repair, approaches compared 55
fluid intake, postoperative care 49
follow-up consultation 53
foot drop, indicator of VVF 3

G
gentamicin 43

H
history-taking 14–15
hydration (preoperative) 19–20
    reasons for 37

I
iatrogenic injury, post-Caesarean intra-
    cervical fistulae 41–2
incidence of VVF 1
incidence of VVF repair 1
infection
    and secondary breakdown 52
    urinary infections 53
instruments 21
intermediate cases 33–43
intra-cervical fistulae 4–6, 40–1
    post-Caesarean 41–2
investigations 18

J

juxta-cervical fistulae 4–6, 12, 36, 39
juxta-urethral fistulae 4, 5, 33–6, 38

K

Katsina methods, *vs* Addis Ababa methods
    55
ketamine 21

L

labial fat grafts for fistula repair 43
lumbar nerves, pressure injury 3

M

methylene blue dye test 17, 29
metronidazole 43
mid-vaginal fistulae 4, 10–11

N

needles 22

O

obstructed labour, ischemic injury sites 3–4
operating table 22
operation (easy case) 24–30
    duration 32
    initial assessment 25
    instruments 21
    lighting 23
    patient position 23–4
    surgeon's position 24
    completion 29–30
        dye test 29
operation (intermediate cases) 33–43
    detached juxta-urethral fistulae 34–6
    detached urethra 34–6
    easy intra-cervical fistulae 40
    scarred juxta-urethral fistulae 33–4
    simple juxta-cervical fistulae 39
    smaller juxta-cervical fistulae 36–8, 40
operation problems/difficulties 31–2
    bladder stones 31–2
    blocked urethra 31
    episiotomies 31
    ureteric involvements 32

P

palpation 16

post-Caesarean intra-cervical fistulae 41–2
post-partum stress 18
postoperative care 46–54
    catheter removal 51–2
    drainage
        blocked catheter 48–9
        closed *vs* open 46–8
    drinking 49
    dryness 50
        causes of wetness 50
    other aspects 50–2
postoperative follow-up 52–3
pre-discharge advice 53
preoperative preparation 19–20
    hydration 19–20
prognosis 7

R

rectal fistulae 18
repair failure, early/late leaks, prognosis
    52

S

sacral nerves, pressure injury 3
scar, amount 7
secondary breakdown, due to infection 52
selection of cases 18
    abominal repair 42
    beginner cases 10–12
    complex cases 12–13
    intermediate cases 33–43
sexual relations 53, 54
stress incontinence
    fibromuscular urethro-vesical sling 35–6
    following complex repairs 53–4
sutures 22

T

tears, lower uterine segment 8
time of fistula repair 9

U

ureteric catheters 37
    substitutes 37
ureteric fistulae 16–18, 42–3
ureteric orifices 37
ureters
    position 37

protection of orifices 37
urethra, blocked 31
urethral catheter, clamping 37
urethral leakage 50
urethral stricture 54
urinary infections 53
uterus
   lower segment tears 8
   rupture, emergency surgery 40

V
vaginal defects, anterior wall 16
vaginal stenosis 16
vault fistulae 40–1
   indications for abdominal surgery 40–1
videos 56–7
VVF
   classification 4
   size 6–7